The Drugs Don't W

Professor Dame Sally C. Davies is the Chief Medical Officer for England and the first woman to hold the post. As CMO she is the independent advisor to the Government on medical matters with particular interest in Public Health and Research. She developed the National Institute for Health Research in 2006. She holds a number of international advisory positions and is an Emeritus Professor at Imperial College.

Dr Jonathan Grant is a Principal Research Fellow and former President at RAND Europe, a not-for-profit public policy research institute. His main research interests are on health R&D policy, and the use of research and evidence in policymaking. He was formerly Head of Policy at The Wellcome Trust. He received his PhD from the Faculty of Medicine, University of London, and his BSc (Econ) from the London School of Economics.

Professor Mike Catchpole is an internationally recognized expert in infectious diseases and the Director of Infectious Disease Surveillance and Control at Public Health England, the government agency charged with protecting and improving health. He has coordinated many national infectious disease outbreak investigations and is an advisor to the European Centre for Disease Prevention and Control. He is also a visiting professor at Imperial College.

The Drugs Don't Work

A Global Threat

Professor Dame Sally C. Davies, Dr Jonathan Grant and Professor Mike Catchpole

VIKING
an imprint of
PENGUIN BOOKS

VIKING

QV
350

Published by the Penguin Group

Penguin Books Ltd, 80 Strand, London WC2R 0RL, England

Penguin Group (USA) Inc., 375 Hudson Street, New York, New York 10014, USA

Penguin Group (Canada), 90 Eglinton Avenue East, Suite 700, Toronto, Ontario,
Canada M4P 2Y3 (a division of Pearson Penguin Canada Inc.)

Penguin Ireland, 25 St Stephen's Green, Dublin 2, Ireland
(a division of Penguin Books Ltd)

Penguin Group (Australia), 707 Collins Street, Melbourne, Victoria 3008, Australia
(a division of Pearson Australia Group Pty Ltd)

Penguin Books India Pvt Ltd, 11 Community Centre,
Panchsheel Park, New Delhi – 110 017, India

Penguin Group (NZ), 67 Apollo Drive, Rosedale, Auckland 0632, New Zealand
(a division of Pearson New Zealand Ltd)

Penguin Books (South Africa) (Pty) Ltd, Block D, Rosebank Office Park,
181 Jan Smuts Avenue, Parktown North, Gauteng 2193, South Africa

Penguin Books Ltd, Registered Offices: 80 Strand, London WC2R 0RL, England

www.penguin.com

First published 2013
001

Copyright © Professor Dame Sally C. Davies, Dr Jonathan Grant
and Professor Mike Catchpole, 2013

The moral right of the contributors has been asserted

Set in 11.75/14pt Dante MT Std
Typeset by Jouve (UK), Milton Keynes
Printed in Great Britain by Clays Ltd, St Ives plc

A CIP catalogue record for this book is available from the British Library

ISBN: 978-0-241-96919-9

www.greenpenguin.co.uk

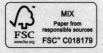

Contents

Introduction

It is a dark July day. Mrs Xu has not been counting, but it is the fifteenth day of her isolation. It started with a wheeze a week after her son's birthday. She had taken Josh to the theme park with a couple of his school friends. She keeps on going back to that day in her mind – it was full of energy and laughter.

The wheeze turned into a cough, the cough into a sore throat. Her husband, Jon, gave her that look – concerned but distant, scared of what was coming. He knew. It had happened to one of his colleagues at work. He was already thinking about what it would mean. How would he look after Josh. Would he cope?

When Josh was born sixteen years ago, the crisis was beginning to take hold. In the final months of her pregnancy, Mrs Xu was advised to stay indoors to separate herself from her friends and family. When Josh went to nursery, she and Jon were lectured by the Head about how irresponsible it was to send a child into public with even mild symptoms. They were given a home testing kit. Josh had to spit on a strip of paper. If it turned green he could attend; if it was red he must stay at home.

They called it 'the red spot'. Jon's mum likened it to a pregnancy test.

A few years later, shortly after Josh joined primary school, the government passed new laws making it a criminal offence for the infected to be in public. There were talks of random tests in the street. If you were contagious, you would be committed to one of the isolation sanatoriums that were being built on the edge of all major towns. This was a death penalty. They were referred to as 'colonies'.

Mrs Xu wants to die at home. She has spent two weeks in her room on her own. Jon and Josh leave her food and medication in the sealed space between the two doors. They use the outer door; she opens the inner door. She speaks to the doctor. He provides her with fever-reducing medicine, painkillers and something to help at the end. He also notifies the authorities. Their home is now identified as an infection spot.

The year is 2043.

As Chief Medical Officer I am the UK government's most senior advisor on health issues. The role dates back to 1855 and I am the sixteenth holder of the post – and the first woman, something that I am immensely proud of. Every year I publish my assessment of the public's health and advise the government on where action is required.

Introduction

In 2012 I decided to focus my first in-depth report on infectious diseases – partly as it seemed to be an uncontroversial topic. I was wrong. I am not easily rattled, but what I learnt scared me – not just as a doctor, but as a mother, a wife and a friend. Breaking from tradition, I engaged the expertise of a broad range of leading clinicians, academics, researchers and policymakers. Our findings were simple:

- We are losing the battle against infectious diseases.
- Bacteria are fighting back and are becoming resistant to modern medicine.
- In short, the drugs don't work.

Since the manufacture of penicillin in 1943, almost all of us have benefited from the medicinal effects of antimicrobial drugs – what we often colloquially and, as we will see, inappropriately refer to as antibiotics. These wonder drugs have stopped us dying from mundane infections such as a sore throat and have allowed us to routinely survive extraordinary operations, from hip replacements to heart transplants. Indeed, the World Health Organization estimates that antimicrobials add, on average, twenty years to everyone's lives. Think about the time your three-year-old child had earache. As an anxious parent you try to console her, but in the early hours of the morning you are at your wits' end and take her to the night clinic, fearing the worst but clinging to the rational best. A five-minute consultation, a prescription, a hunt for the open pharmacy and you are home with a fluorescent yellow medicine. Twenty-four hours later your loved one is playing in the garden oblivious to the drama of the night before.

The story of Mrs Xu may read like science fiction, or a scenario from *World War Z*, but if we do not change the course of history, and if we allow resistance to increase, in a few decades we may start dying from the most commonplace of ailments that can today be treated easily. We will regress to the point where, in twenty years' time, when I need a hip replacement, the operation may be deemed too dangerous to even attempt due to the risk of catching an untreatable infection.

Antimicrobial drugs have been important to me. In the late 1970s, my husband, Philip, was diagnosed with chronic myeloid leukaemia (CML). The only treatment available for CML at that time was symptomatic, but colleagues had developed a new way of extending life: they collected the stem cells circulating in his blood early in his disease and froze them. In this way, they could be given back to him when, as always happens, his chronic leukaemia developed into the lethal, acute form.

In 1980, Philip's CML transformed into acute leukaemia – his death sentence. Naturally, we wanted more time together. He was given very high doses of chemotherapy to kill the leukaemia cells, and began the stem cell transfusion. The hope was that the stem cells (or bone marrow) would produce both CML and normal blood cells. With a transplant of this kind, the bone marrow can take days or weeks to regenerate and then to take effect. In the intervening period, patients have to be supported with red blood cell transfusions, platelets to prevent bleeding and antimicrobial drugs to thwart and treat infection. This is an awful time for everyone: there was a chance that Philip could die of bleeding or infection before his transfused cells settled in and grew back. Every day we anxiously checked for bruises indicating bleeding and his temperature chart for infection. He was assaulted with swabs and needles at the whiff of a rise in temperature; the best care he could receive, but extremely stressful.

The first time Philip received this course of treatment he lasted three months before the acute leukaemia returned. The second time was even shorter, and after the third time the severe form of the disease was detected in his blood at the same time as the normal blood cells were returning. He declined further treatments, but thanks to a combination of stem cell rescue and antimicrobials he was granted nearly an extra year of life with me. This was very special for both of us.

Patients with low or absent white cells, or poor

immunity, such as Philip or people receiving strong anti-cancer treatment, receive essential intravenous antimicrobial drugs as life-saving measures. They are supported by a number of other measures to prevent the introduction of infectious agents, including staying in an isolation room, very strict hand-washing, disinfection and meticulous mouth care, including rather horrid-tasting antiseptic mouthwashes. It is clear, however, that none of these treatments would be successful without antibacterials, antifungals and antivirals, used both to prevent infection and to treat infections as they occur. My mother, during treatment for ovarian cancer, depended on antimicrobials to endure her stronger treatments.

But the power of these drugs may be coming to an end. We have taken antibacterial and other antimicrobial drugs for granted for too long. We have misused them through overuse and false prescription, and as a result the bugs are growing in resistance and fighting back. We are also not developing new drugs fast enough. This is not a distant threat: already, resistant bugs are killing 25,000 people a year across Europe. That is almost the same number as die in road traffic accidents.

My intention in this book is to draw attention to this potentially devastating story. I am joined in this endeavour by my two colleagues: a policy and research expert, Dr Jonathan Grant, and an infectious disease epidemiologist, Professor Mike Catchpole. Jonathan is a long-time and trusted advisor and esteemed analyst who works at RAND Europe, a research organization that aims to improve public policy. Mike is an internationally recognized expert in infectious diseases and the Director of the Centre for Infectious Disease Surveillance and Control at Public Health England, the government agency charged with protecting and improving our health.

In the following chapters we attempt to provide a scientific overview of microbes and how they can cause human disease. We identify different treatment options and examine how the rules of evolution mean the bugs are constantly adapting to those treatments. But more importantly we explain what can be done about it, from changes in personal hygiene to developing new drugs.

Our response needs to be global and multifaceted, but if we do work together, bringing the ingenuity of humanity to this real, growing and often forgotten global threat, we can manage and mitigate the risk of antimicrobial resistance, which is just as important and deadly as climate change and international terrorism.

1.

Man, Microbes and Microbiomes

'If it is a terrifying thought that life is at the mercy of the multiplication of these minute bodies, it is a consoling hope that science will not always remain powerless before such enemies . . .'

Louis Pasteur,
paper read to the French Academy of Sciences, 1878

Infections have dominated the history of human disease, and at times they have dominated history itself. The Black Death swept across the world in the fourteenth century, from its probable origins in China to its peak in Europe, where it reduced the population by an estimated 30–60 per cent. In 1918 the influenza pandemic, sometimes referred to as the 'Spanish flu', is estimated to have killed at least 50 million people worldwide. It is this potential for infectious diseases to spread rapidly from human, animal or environmental sources, and thereby give rise to outbreaks, epidemics or even pandemics that circle the globe, that makes them a unique threat. On a global scale, infections are still the leading cause of human morbidity and mortality, particularly because of their impact on lower-income countries such as in Africa and South East Asia, but also because of the long-term disability that they can cause in richer countries, through healthcare-associated infections and the consequences of viral infections such as hepatitis C and HIV.

Antimicrobials are a group of drugs that provide us with the weapons to fight these (still) important causes of disease, disability and death. Their discovery and use through the second half of the twentieth century has had a profound effect on human health and has been essential to modern medical advances such as the treatment of cancer. We are now, however, at a crossroads in the journey towards the defeat of infection as a cause of disease, as our use of these valuable drugs is not only becoming threatened by the spectre of resistance among the bugs they are used to treat, but also as we recognize that their injudicious use can cause harm in its own right.

Infectious diseases are caused by minute organisms that can be found living in or on plants and animals, and also in the inanimate environment, such as in water and soil. These minute organisms range from viruses and bacteria, to fungi and protozoans (and infections may also be caused by larger multicellular organisms such as parasitic worms). Although the majority of these microbes are too small to be seen with the naked eye, and they lack the complexity of higher life forms, they nevertheless share with humans and other animals many of the building blocks for life, such as ribonucleic acid (RNA) or deoxyribonucleic acid (DNA) for coding of genetic information and protein-based structural and functional elements. This sharing of building blocks limits the opportunities for treatment, since treatments need to be able to kill the microbes by interfering with their structure or metabolism, but not with the cells of the human (or animal, fish, insect, plant, etc.) that they are infecting.

The relationship between man and microbes, particularly bacteria, is complex. While bacteria are an important cause of infectious disease, the great majority of the enormous number of bacteria that we carry around with us as normal healthy individuals are harmless passengers ('commensals'), or even benefit the hosts that harbour them, as long as they remain where they are normally found, which is mainly in the gut and on the skin. These commensal bacteria help to keep our bodies healthy by aiding in the digestion of foods and by producing vitamins B and K, which we can absorb. They also play a role in the development of the immune system and inhibit the growth of harmful bacteria that can cause disease, by competing with them. The beneficial roles of bacteria that occur naturally as part of the human biome ('good bacteria') are often given as the rationale for the use of probiotics. These are live microbes that are the same as, or similar to, those found naturally in the human body. Probiotics are often found in products such as dietary supplements, yoghurts and suppositories. A 2008 overview of clinical applications of probiotics published in the journal *Clinical Infectious Diseases* concluded that strong evidence exists for their benefit in the management of acute and antibacterial-associated diarrhoea, and substantial evidence exists for their having a beneficial effect in atopic eczema (a skin condition most commonly seen in infants). Commensal bacteria in the vagina are also important in inhibiting the growth of bacteria that can cause infection of the newborn baby as it passes through the birth canal.

The term given to describe the entirety of microorganisms that reside in or on the human body is the human microbiome. It has been estimated that the microorganisms in the human microbiome outnumber the cells that make up the human body by 10 to 1, and that as such each human carries around 100 trillion (10^{14}) microorganisms. Some of the microorganisms cause illnesses, but many are necessary for good health. Researchers now calculate that around 1,000 different bacterial species can be found within the human intestine alone, and that the total weight of bacteria within the human gut can be as much as 2kg.

Large as it may be, the human microbiome is only a small part of the total of all microorganisms that live on the Earth. There are approximately 5×10^{30} bacteria on Earth, making up a biomass that equals or exceeds that of all plants and animals on Earth, and containing ten times the quantity of nutrients found in plants and animals. Most of these microorganisms live in the soil, the open ocean and on the ocean floor. There are typically 40 million bacterial cells in a gram of soil and a million bacterial cells in a millilitre of fresh water.

The time that it takes for bacterial cells (or populations) to divide, and therefore spread, is called the generation time. This time varies considerably between bacterial species and according to the environment within which the bacteria are growing. The rate of cell replication for all prokaryotes (all bacteria and other organisms that lack a nucleus) on Earth is estimated at 1.7×10^{30} cells every year. The enormous size of this population and the speed with which its members replicate provide a huge capacity for genetic diversity. The generation time for a prokaryote such as *Escherichia coli* (E. coli) in the intestinal tract is estimated to be twelve to twenty-four hours, although under optimal conditions in a laboratory it can be as short as fifteen to twenty minutes (compared to a generation time of between twenty and thirty years for most human populations, i.e. the mean age of mothers at first childbirth).

Microbes and microbial disease

Microbes can cause a wide range of diseases, reflecting the many different ways in which they interact with and affect the host they are infecting. Disease may stem from the direct action of the microbe on the host's cells, or from the inferred action of toxins released by the microbe. It may also be caused by the host's own immune response to the infection (Table 1).

Table 1: Different ways microbes can cause diseases

MECHANISM OF ACTION	EXAMPLES
Killing of the host's cells by invading microbes	Killing of cells in the host's respiratory system by influenza, leading to flu and pneumonia
	Killing of cells in the host's central nervous system by poliovirus, leading to paralysis
Interference with host cell functions by microbial toxins	Tetanus and botulism bacteria both cause disease by the release of toxins that interfere with the nervous system control of muscles
	Cholera bacterium causes the release of toxins that promote excessive secretion of fluids by the cells of the gut
Modification of host cell behaviour	The human papilloma virus inhibits tumour suppressor pathways in infected host cells, causing cancer
Disease symptoms and signs caused by the host's immune response	Cell damage caused by the host's immune response to tuberculosis and hepatitis A

An understanding of the structure and functioning of microbes is critically important to our understanding of how they can infect humans (and other animals) and cause disease, and also to how drugs can be developed and used to treat the diseases that they cause. This next section provides a brief description of the main types of microbe that this book will focus upon, before we go on to describe how we can use drugs to treat the infections that they cause.

Viruses are the smallest of the microbial life forms, and have a relatively simple structure that consists mainly of a genome (the genetic code) made up of either DNA or RNA, which is contained within an outer coat made up of proteins, and sometimes also fat molecules (known as lipids). The genome carries the code that allows the virus to replicate and multiply once it has invaded a host's cell, while the outer coat protects the genome from the surrounding environment and enables the virus to bind to the walls of the cells that they infect. Viruses may also contain other proteins (enzymes) that are required for the initial steps in replication of the virus when it infects a cell. While some viruses can survive in the environment, sometimes in relatively harsh conditions, all viruses can replicate only within the living cells of a host organism that they have infected, making use of the host cell's systems to produce copies of themselves. The fact that viruses cannot replicate other than by using the 'machinery' of the cells of the animal, or plant, that they infect not only challenges our concepts of what constitutes a life form, but also limits the targets that we can direct drugs against. Nonetheless, viruses have the essential characteristics of being able to invade cells, to reproduce and respond to evolutionary pressures, and the limited structural components that they need in order to achieve those basic behaviours can be exploited as targets for drug treatment.

Bacteria are single-celled microorganisms that are typically about one-tenth the size of the cells that make up most of the human body. Bacteria consist of a chromosome made of DNA that is enclosed, along with other intracellular components, within a membrane that is made up of lipids and proteins. Bacteria may also contain genetic code in plasmids, which are usually small, circular loops of DNA that can be found floating free in the interior of bacteria, but are separate from the main bacterial chromosome, and may carry genes that are important to the ability of the bacteria to cause disease or to survive under hostile conditions. Plasmids are important because they can be transferred between bacteria of different species, as well as between bacteria of the same species. Unlike viruses, bacteria also possess a range of other structural and functional components that are important to their survival and their ability to replicate, which offer potential targets for anti-microbial drugs. The great majority of bacteria also have a cell wall, made up of sugars and amino acids, that is located outside the cell membrane and provides structural support and protection. The cell wall, which is not found in humans or other animals, is essential to the survival of many bacteria, and differences in the detailed structure of the cell wall can have an important effect on how susceptible bacteria are to antibacterial drugs. Bacteria are often classified broadly according to how their cell wall reacts to a particular staining agent (the Gram stain) when viewed under a microscope, with Gram-positive bacteria staining blue and exhibiting different susceptibilities to certain common antibacterials than the Gram-negative bacteria, which appear red, as a result of picking up a counter-stain.

Fungi are a large group of organisms that are considered to be distinct from animals and plants (and from viruses and bacteria). They range from large structures, such as mushrooms, to microscopic structures, which include microorganisms that can infect humans – such as athlete's foot – other animals and plants. Fungi possess chromosomes that are composed of DNA located within a distinct nucleus within the fungal cell, and may replicate through sexual or asexual reproduction. Fungi, like bacteria (and plants), possess a cell wall, although its composition is different from that of bacteria.

Antimicrobials and antimicrobial treatment

Our first line of defences against infection are the physical barriers that the body has to prevent microbial invasion. These include an intact covering of skin, the acid that we have in our stomachs, and the microscopic hair-like structures in our airways that push any potential invading organisms out of our lungs.

When these natural defences are breached, because the invading microorganism is particularly virulent or our defences have been weakened by disease, injury or medical treatment, we have another line of defence at the ready. Many infections, particularly viral ones, are effectively dealt with by the body's chemical defence systems – such as lysozyme, found in tears and saliva – which attack the cell wall of bacteria, and specialized proteins in the blood (the 'complement' system) that can attack microbes and attract immune cells. These immune cells not only help to defend the body against current infection, but also often provide us with long-term immunity to future infection by the same strain of microbe. However, in some circumstances antimicrobial drugs may be required.

Drugs that kill or inhibit the growth of microbes have been the mainstay of therapy for infectious disease since the introduction of penicillin for treating infection in the 1940s. It is astonishing to think that the discovery of this wonder drug was accidental. When was the last time you went to the kitchen for a slice of toast and noticed a number of small fuzzy spots of mould on your bread? Chances are you had been away for a few days and forgot to give the bread and other perishables to your neighbours or friends before you left. It happens to us all, but we don't win Nobel prizes on the back of such mistakes. Alexander Fleming did. Born in 1881 in Ayrshire, Scotland, he had moved to London when he was sixteen and ended up studying medicine at St Mary's Hospital after a few clerical jobs and a generous inheritance. At medical school he was a couple of years older than his contemporaries, and aided by this maturity and his sharp intellect he won many student prizes. On the surface Fleming was dour and unassuming, but his interests pointed to a more complex personality: he was a Freemason, a member of the Chelsea Arts Club, a private in the London Scottish Regiment and a first-rate shot for St Mary's Hospital rifle club. Partly influenced by concerns that Fleming could end up shooting for a rival hospital team, he was offered a job as an assistant in St Mary's Inoculation Department in 1906. He qualified as a doctor a few years later and began to develop a reputation as a 'pox doctor', treating sexually transmitted diseases both in the poorhouses of West London and through a lucrative private practice. But the outbreak of war was to change that. In October 1914 Fleming joined colleagues from the Inoculation Department in establishing an army laboratory for the study of wound infections at Boulogne, France. Gangrene and tetanus would be responsible for nearly a tenth of all deaths in field hospitals during the First World War. Fleming wanted to understand the cause of these infections, and found that the majority of them were coming from the soldiers' own clothing. He investigated the effects of antiseptic washing, which was the standard treatment at the time, and found it to be potentially counterproductive, especially for the deep wounds typically inflicted in war. Bacteria arising from a wound were attacked by the body's own white bloods cells (phagocytes), but they themselves were being killed off by the antiseptics, allowing the bacteria to flourish.

Flem – as his colleagues called him – was demobilized in 1919 and returned to the Inoculation Department at St Mary's as an acknowledged expert on wound infection. His research interests over the next ten years were largely focused around lysozyme – a natural enzyme that acts like an antiseptic, providing protection from some bacteria – which he discovered in 1921.

In the summer of 1928, Fleming went on holiday with his wife Sareen and four-year-old son, Robert. They had bought a country home, The Dhoon, in the picturesque Suffolk village of Barton Mill in 1921, and spent most of their holidays and weekends there. On returning to his laboratory in London at the beginning of September he discovered that the Petri dishes he had left on his bench had gone mouldy. He was investigating the properties of *Staphylococcus aureus*, a common bacterium that can cause skin infections such as boils. As was typical of Fleming, he had not cleaned or tidied his lab before going on holiday, creating an ideal environment for the mould to fester. What perplexed Fleming was not the growth of the mould but that the mould seemed to have killed off the bacteria that he was growing in the cultures. Intrigued by this observation, he set about identifying the mould and discovered it was *Penicillium*, a common and naturally occurring genus of fungi that had first been described at the beginning of the nineteenth century. He managed to purify the 'mould juice' and test it against a number of known bacteria that cause common diseases such as diphtheria, pneumonia and meningitis. Fleming reproduced the results of the accidental experiment and called the antibacterial 'penicillin', publishing his findings in the *Journal of Experimental Pathology* in 1929.

Convinced that he had discovered one of the world's foremost blockbuster drugs, Fleming spent subsequent years trying to purify and isolate the antibacterial properties of penicillin and demonstrate its clinical value. He failed and had given up when two Oxford chemists – Ernst Chain and Howard Florey – took up this challenge in the late 1930s. At the time their interest was academic: 'The possibility that penicillin could have practical use in clinical medicine did not enter our minds when we started the work,' Chain said later in life. They succeeded in developing a way to isolate, purify and produce small quantities of penicillin. In May 1940 they tested the drug on eight white mice by injecting them with large amounts of streptococci. Four mice were left untreated: the 'control' group, and the other four injected with different doses of penicillin. The mice in the control group died within a couple of hours, while the treated mice survived. They had managed to demonstrate the potential clinical application of penicillin when war was beginning to rage around Europe. The animal experiment was followed by a successful toxicology test in a healthy volunteer in 1941 and a series of clinical trials, so that in 1942 the General Penicillin Committee was set up to coordinate commercial production as part of the war effort. Glaxo, a drug company, established a penicillin production plant in Britain in December 1942, but it was difficult for the British companies to ramp up production given their existing commitments for other medicines. Florey managed to persuade the US government to fund the equipment for drug companies to mass-produce penicillin in America. By 1944 there was enough penicillin to be given routinely to all wounded soldiers, and it was seen as the original 'wonder drug' at a time when good news was rare. In recognition 'for the discovery of penicillin and its curative effect in various infectious diseases', Fleming, Chain and Florey jointly won the Nobel Prize in Physiology or Medicine in 1945.

There is often confusion about the terms used to describe drugs that are effective against microbes. The common unifying term for all these drugs is 'antimicrobials' (although 'antibiotic' is often used as the colloquial equivalent). The term 'antibiotic' was first used in 1942 to describe substances that are produced naturally by microbes and that inhibit the growth of, or kill, other microbes. These substances provide the microbes that produce them with a competitive advantage, and hence enable them to flourish, over the microbes that they inhibit or kill through the release of antibiotic substances. In strict scientific terms, this means that we should not describe as antibiotics the many drugs that are partially or wholly manufactured through man-made chemical processes, and that we now use to treat infections, as they are not produced by microbes. The language of drug treatment for infections is further complicated by the fact that the great majority of such drugs are active only against viruses, or bacteria, or fungi (or other causes of infection). This leads to the use of terms such as 'antiviral', 'antibacterial' and 'antifungal' for the different classes of drug that we use.

We will use 'antimicrobial' as the general term to describe all drugs that are used to treat microbial infections, and 'antibacterial', 'antiviral' and 'antifungal' when we are discussing drugs that are used primarily to treat forms of infection caused by bacteria, viruses or fungi respectively. Within those groupings, the drugs may also be classified according to their underlying mode of action or their effect on the microorganism they are being used against, for example bacteriostatic (only inhibit bacterial growth) or bacteriocidal (kill bacteria). Different types of viruses, bacteria and fungi are susceptible to different types of antimicrobial drug, and different strains of the same type of virus, bacteria or fungi can differ in which drugs they are susceptible to (because they can acquire resistance). As with any drug, antimicrobial drugs can give rise to adverse reactions (sometimes called 'side effects'), which in rare cases can be severe. For this reason, and because of the risks of promoting antimicrobial resistance through inappropriate use of drugs, it is important that antimicrobials are only used when they are likely to be of benefit in the treatment of an infection, which means knowing which infection and which antimicrobials that strain of infection is likely to be susceptible to.

Unfortunately, it is often not possible to be certain whether the illness in a patient with infectious disease is viral, bacterial, or due to another form of microbe, without undertaking laboratory tests. Thus, in the majority of cases, it is not possible for a doctor to know with certainty whether a patient with a sore throat has a bacterial form of infection that might benefit from antibacterial treatment, let alone which form of bacterial infection and hence which type of antibacterial drug would be of benefit. Indeed, if the patient has a viral form of infection then antibacterial treatment would be of no help whatsoever. In most causes of viral sore throat, antiviral treatment would not be of use either, as currently available antiviral drugs are not effective against the majority of common causes of the ailment. Furthermore, these common causes of viral throat infection are effectively eliminated over time by a normal body's immune system.

Antimicrobial treatment, particularly repeated courses and treatment with broad-spectrum antibacterials, can, in addition to eliminating the harmful bacteria causing disease, also substantially reduce the number of the commensal bacteria that live in and on our bodies. In the case of the commensals that live in our intestines, this can lead to the gut being colonized with harmful bacteria in their place. Indeed, the use of broad-spectrum antimicrobials is now recognized as a major factor behind the rise in a serious form of infection of the intestine called *Clostridium difficile*, towards the end of the twentieth century and the beginning of this one. As we will see, this has become one of the most important causes of infection affecting patients in hospital, and in 2011 *Clostridium difficile* was mentioned on the death certificates of just over 2,300 people in the UK. The good news is that the number of cases and deaths due to this infection has declined dramatically as a result of the introduction of strict controls on the use of antimicrobials in hospital and the reintroduction of strong infection control measures including handwashing.

The challenge in developing new drugs for systemic use is to find substances that are active against microbial cell structures and metabolic processes but not against structures and processes in the cells of the human patient who is to receive the treatment. This is why many of the drugs we use today to treat bacterial infections target the cell wall, which exists in most bacteria but not in humans. Examples of such drugs include the penicillins, as listed in the Appendix. Other targets for antibacterial drugs include the bacterial cell membrane, bacterial protein production, and bacterial DNA replication and/or transcription. Some antibacterial drugs are active against a wide range of bacteria, such as the carbapenems and tetracyclines, whereas others have a much narrower spectrum of activity, such as vancomycin, which is only effective at killing sensitive Gram-positive bacteria. Metronidazole, which acts by inactivating a wide range of enzymes, is active against a range of bacteria and also against protozoal infections (which, for example, can cause amoebic dysentery).

Most of today's antibacterial drugs are man-made (semi-synthetic) modifications of naturally occurring compounds. These include, for example, the penicillins (which were originally identified as a compound produced by *Penicillium* fungi). Some antibacterial compounds are still isolated from living organisms, such as the group of antibiotics that are called aminoglycosides, which are usually used only for treating severe infections in hospitalized patients as their blood levels need to be monitored closely to avoid the hearing and kidney damage that can be caused if levels become too high. Others, such as the sulphonamides, are produced solely by chemical synthesis.

As with antibacterial drugs, antiviral drugs target viral components or processes that are as distinct as possible from human cell components and processes. The earliest antiviral drugs in wide use were those developed against influenza (amantadine) and herpes viruses (acyclovir), although the major focus of antiviral drug development in more recent years has been with respect to HIV infection. Antiviral drugs work by targeting key steps in the stages of invasion of the host cell, replication of the viral genome, and assembly and release of the new virus once the genome has been replicated. For example, amantadine, which is used in the treatment of influenza, inhibits the step of uncoating the viral genome that is necessary for the virus's genetic code to be inserted into the host's cells so that it can be replicated. Acyclovir, used for the treatment of herpes virus infections, many of the drugs used for the treatment of HIV infection, and lamivudine, used for the treatment of hepatitis B, all work by inhibiting the replication of the virus after invasion of the host cell. Oseltamivir, another drug used for the treatment of influenza, works by inhibiting the release of the virus from the host cell after it has been replicated.

There are greater similarities between fungal and human cells at the molecular level than there are between human cells and either viruses or bacterial cells. As a consequence, identifying targets for drugs in the treatment of fungal infections has proved more difficult, and side effects from systemic anti-fungal drugs are more common. Many of the drugs used for treating systemic fungal infections target the cell membrane, which contains ergosterol in place of the cholesterol component found in human cell membranes.

2.

The Fall and Rise of Infection

'The time may come when penicillin can be bought by anyone in the shops. Then there is the danger that the ignorant man may easily underdose himself and by exposing his microbes to non-lethal quantities of the drug make them resistant. Here is a hypothetical illustration. Mr X has a sore throat. He buys some penicillin and gives himself, not enough to kill the streptococci but enough to educate them to resist penicillin. He then infects his wife. Mrs X gets pneumonia and is treated with penicillin. As the streptococci are now resistant to penicillin the treatment fails. Mrs X dies. Who is primarily responsible for Mrs X's death?'

Sir Alexander Fleming,
Nobel Lecture, 1945

From happy accident to global blockbuster

Sixteen years passed between Sir Alexander Fleming's accidental discovery of pencillin in 1928 and its mass production in 1943. Penicillin became a life saver in the Second World War because Sir Howard Florey and Sir Ernst Chain helped turn it into a useable drug. But it was the expertise of American drug companies that allowed the wonder drug to be mass-produced. They succeeded in making large quantities of penicillin using a technique known as deep-tank fermentation, where the anti-bacterial drug was grown in large quantities in an aerobic mixture of corn steep liquor, milk sugar, salts and minerals, which controlled for pH and the sterility of the air. Due to these changes in manufacturing techniques, output increased exponentially from 21 billion Oxford units in 1943 to 6.8 trillion in 1945. (An Oxford unit is the minimum amount of penicillin that will prevent the growth of *Staphylococcus aureus* over an area an inch in diameter in a standard culture medium and is equivalent to 0.606 micrograms of the crystalline compound – a typical dose of benzylpenicillin for an adult with a throat or skin infection caused by sensitive Gram-positive bacteria today would be 4 to 8 million units per day.) The American government was able to remove all restrictions on penicillin in 1945, and in the UK it first became available to the general public as a prescription drug a year later.

Today over 35 million courses of antimicrobial drugs are prescribed by family doctors in England each year – that's more than one prescription per household per year. Millions of doses of antimicrobials are given in hospitals each day, with prophylactic use of antibacterials before surgery now a routine precaution for many types of operation. When compared to other European countries, the UK is not a major consumer of antimicrobial drugs. European Surveillance of Antimicrobial Consumption is an international network that collects comparable and reliable use data. They estimate the 'defined daily dose' (DDD) per 1,000 people for antimicrobial drugs. The DDD is an international accepted statistical measure that helps to make comparisons between countries. Actual doses for individual patients and patient groups will often differ from the DDD. In 2009, the latest the data are available, the DDD for outpatient antimicrobial consumption in the UK was 17 for every 1,000 people, which was about average for Europe. By comparison, the DDD for Greece was nearly twice that, at 38. Cyprus, France, Italy, Luxembourg and Belgium all had comparatively high rates of antimicrobial consumption. One of the reasons for these large differences in prescribing practice is the availability of antimicrobial drugs from pharmacists. By contrast to the UK, where the availability of antimicrobial drugs is strictly controlled through the need for a prescription from a qualified doctor or a pharmacist, in some countries you can buy them over the counter. (The only exception in the UK is for the issuing of single doses of azithromycin by pharmacists for the treatment of a laboratory-confirmed chlamydia infection, and the over-the-counter availability of two of the antimicrobials used as prophylactics against malaria.)

Researchers in Catalonia, Spain, asked two actors to visit nearly 200 pharmacies. The actors pretended they had either a sore throat, acute bronchitis or a urinary tract infection. Antibacterial drugs were sold without prescription in nearly half of the cases, although it did depend a bit on the condition, ranging from around 17 per cent for the sore throat to 80 per cent for the urinary tract infection. Another study in the UK found that nearly 6 per cent of households had antimicrobial drugs in their medicine cabinets, unused from a previous prescription. Half of these households had kept them in case of future illness. This is doubly worrying, as it indicates that people may not be completing their prescription and that they plan to self-medicate with a likely incomplete course of medication – both of which increase the risk of colonization and infection with drug-resistant organisms.

But the use and misuse of antimicrobial drugs is not restricted to humans. Globally the vast majority of antimicrobial drugs are given to farmed animals, including cattle, sheep, chickens and pigs. Like humans, sick animals can be treated with the drugs, but they are also used prophylactically in animals at high risk, such as those intensively farmed. In the UK, a total of 447 tonnes of anti-microbials were sold for animal use in 2010, of which 87 per cent were purchased for prophylaxis and treatment of infections in food-producing animals. More controversially, antimicrobials are sometimes used to fatten them up for slaughter – a side effect of antimicrobial use. They are also routinely used in plant agriculture – for example in spraying fruit – and even as antifungal paints on ships, oil pipes and for other industrial uses.

The fall of infection

In 2011, 55 million people died out of a global population of 6.9 billion. About 10 million, roughly a fifth, of these deaths were from infectious diseases: 9.5 million from low- and middle-income countries and half a million from high-income countries. Put another way, 40 per cent of all deaths in low-income countries were a result of infectious diseases, compared to around 7 per cent in the UK and other high-income countries. If you include illness in these estimates, then infections resulted in the loss of 564 million disability-adjusted life years in 2010, just under a quarter of the global burden of disease. A disability-adjusted life year (or DALY) is a composite measure that combines the time lost due to premature death with the time of healthy life lost due to illness. In high-income countries the burden of infectious diseases is relatively low – at less than one-twentieth of all DALYs – but in low-income countries (particularly those in sub-Saharan Africa), by contrast, infectious diseases account for at least one-third of DALYs.

Over the past 100 years, many high-income countries have experienced a significant decline in death rates. Life expectancy has rapidly increased during this time. For instance, life expectancy at birth in the UK was just below fifty years in 1900, sixty-eight years in 1950 and eighty years in 2010. As illustrated in Figure 1 (below), death rates fell three-fold, from 16,958 deaths for every million people in the UK in 1901 to around 5,384 in 1971 (these figures are standardized for age and sex, so they are not distorted by changes in the age structure of the population). About three-quarters of this decline is due to a drop in infectious diseases: the death rate for infectious diseases fell nine-fold, from 9,346 to 1,111 deaths for every million people between 1901 and 1971.

If you look at specific causes of death, then the statistics are more dramatic. Deaths from puerperal fever (infection after childbirth) in the early 1930s were 1,000–1,200 deaths per 1,000,000 live births, despite rigorous hygienic precautions, but within ten years of the introduction of sulphona-mides in the 1930s, and subsequently of penicillin in the 1940s, this rate fell to almost zero. Likewise, deaths from syphilis all but disappeared in the twentieth century. Although these declines in mortality coincided with the introduction of anti-microbial drugs, it would be wrong to attribute all or even the majority of this health gain to the won-der drugs. Almost without exception, the decline in deaths from the biggest killers at the beginning of the twentieth century predates the introduction of antimicrobial drugs for civilian use at the end of the Second World War. Just over half of the decline in infectious diseases had occurred before 1931. The main influences on the decline in mortal-ity were better nutrition, improved hygiene and sanitation, and less dense housing, which all helped to prevent and to reduce transmission of infectious diseases.

These broader environmental influences of poor sanitation, overcrowding and malnutrition partly explain why infectious disease is still a major cause of death and illness in low- and middle-income countries. For low-income countries, life expect-ancy is currently about sixty years. Pneumonia and diarrhoeal diseases currently account for a third of

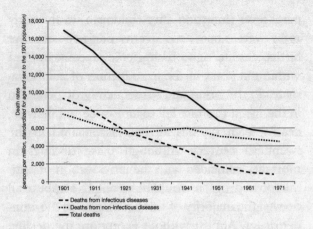

Figure 1: Age-standardized death rates by cause of death,
England and Wales, 1901–1971

Source: McKeown et al., 1975

all deaths to children under the age of five, with the highest burden occurring in Africa and South East Asia. But there is a glimmer of hope that infectious disease in the world's poorer countries is beginning to be controlled. For example, childhood immunization against measles has increased. In 1990 about three-quarters of all children globally had received a vaccination; by 2009, coverage was 83 per cent, with low-income countries experiencing the highest increase. Likewise, a number of countries have recorded decreases in the number of confirmed cases of malaria since 2000. Globally the estimated number of deaths from malaria fell from almost 1 million in

2000 to 781,000 in 2009. In Africa there was a reduction of more than 50 per cent in either confirmed
malaria cases or malaria admissions and deaths over
the same period. However, the number of people living with HIV worldwide continues to grow, reaching
an estimated 33.3 million people in 2009 – 23 per cent
higher than in 1999. That said, the overall growth of
the global epidemic appears to have stabilized; in
2009, the estimated number of new HIV infections
was 19 per cent lower than in 1999. The increasing
number of people living with HIV reflects in part the
life-prolonging effects of antiretroviral therapy.
According to the World Health Organization, as of
December 2009, antiretroviral therapy was available to more than 5 million people in low-income
and middle-income countries, although coverage
remained low, with only one-third of people with
HIV receiving this treatment.

For over three generations, Europe and North
America have experienced an extraordinary and
unprecedented decline in mortality. The world's
poorer regions are beginning to experience this
demographic transition but still have unacceptably
high levels of avoidable death and illness. The
cause of the decline in the world's rich countries
and the persistent inequity in poor countries is due
to a combination of economic development and
access to modern medicine. We have the tools to win
the battle against infectious diseases. Unfortunately,

these actual and potential gains are under threat. The antimicrobial drugs that have helped combat infectious diseases are becoming less and less effective.

The rise of the resistant bug

The same bacteria that Fleming was investigating when he discovered penicillin – *Staphylococcus aureus* – became resistant to the drug in the 1950s. *Staphylococcus aureus* is a common cause of skin infection, respiratory diseases and food poisoning. To address the penicillin-resistant *Staphylococcus aureus*, methicillin – a new class of antimicrobial drugs – was developed in the 1960s. Methicillin-resistant *Staphylococcus aureus* (MRSA) emerged quite quickly but became headline news in the 1990s following a number of high-profile cases of people catching the infection in hospitals.

Bacteria can be considered promiscuous in that they have developed several different ways of sharing their genetic material, facilitating the ease and speed of evolution of drug-resistant strains. The most common is by passing genes from mother to daughter, as we all do through our family lineage. Secondly, bacteria are also able to exchange genetic material in the form of plasmid DNA that exists separately from the main chromosomal DNA, and which may include the genetic code for antimicrobial resistance. Plasmids may be exchanged not only 'vertically', to 'daughter' bacteria, through the process of bacterial replication by division, but also 'horizontally', through contact with other bacteria. Importantly, this exchange can occur not only between members of the same bacterial species, but also between different bacterial species. In this way resistance that has been developed or acquired by one strain of bacteria, including strains that are found as normal commensals in the human gut, can be spread to other strains or species, including strains and species that can cause severe disease. (In some cases the plasmid DNA can become incorporated into the main bacterial chromosomal DNA.) Thirdly, bacteria can also acquire new genetic material, including genes for antimicrobial resistance, by taking up exogenous DNA from their environment, in a process called transformation, or as a result of being infected by a form of virus that is called a bacteriophage, which can introduce foreign DNA into the chromosome.

Genes for resistance can exert their effect through any of five broad types of mechanism: (i) the bacteria can inactivate the drug before it reaches its target within the bacterial cell; (ii) the outer layers of the cell can be impermeable, and prevent the drug from entering; (iii) the drug can enter but is then pumped back out again ('efflux');

(iv) the target can be altered so that it is no longer recognized by the antibacterial; or (v) the bacteria can acquire an alternative metabolic pathway that renders the antibacterial's target redundant ('bypass'). Although some hundreds of resistances are known, virtually all can be ascribed to one of these five broad types of mechanism.

There are now examples of drug-resistant strains in all types of microorganisms, including bacteria (e.g. *Staphylococcus aureus*), viruses (HIV and hepatitis B), fungi and parasites (malaria). Antimicrobial resistance in hospitals and other healthcare settings presents a particular threat. This is because of the inevitably high use of antimicrobial drugs in healthcare settings and the ease of patient-to-patient transmission. It is estimated that about 4 million patients acquire a healthcare-associated infection in the European Union every year. Drug-resistant bacteria are responsible for about 25,000 deaths a year, which translate into healthcare costs and productivity losses of €1.5 billion annually in the EU. In England in 2011, there were 1,185 reported cases of MRSA, but this had declined from a peak of 7,700 cases eight years earlier. This success was largely due to public and political pressure in improving hospital infection control, including mandatory reporting, infection reduction targets and 'deep cleans' of infected wards.

As we perhaps begin to get to grips with MRSA, new challenges begin to emerge, such as *Escherichia coli* (E. coli). E. coli is a bacterium that is found in large numbers in the lower intestine and is normally harmless, but certain types can cause serious food poisoning and it is the most frequent cause of bloodstream infection in European hospitals. In the UK in 2011, over 100,000 cases of bloodstream infection were reported to the Health Protection Agency. E. coli alone accounted for around 36 per cent of these, compared with 11 per cent for *Staphylococcus aureus* (of which just 1.6 per cent were due to MRSA). Recent European data suggest a 30 per cent mortality for patients with septicaemia due to multi-resistant E. coli, compared with 15 per cent for those with susceptible E. coli.

But healthcare-acquired infections are not a rich-country problem. Recent analysis by the World Health Organization found that healthcare-associated infections are more frequent in resource-limited settings than in developed countries. For every 100 hospitalized patients, around 10 will catch an infection in developing countries, compared to around 7 in high-income countries. About one-third of operated patients will catch an infection following surgery, which is nine times higher than in developed countries. Healthcare facilities in developing countries provide the perfect environment for the transmission of resistant bugs. In addition to those factors evident in developed countries – Darwinian selection and patient-to-patient transmission – there is a limited spectrum of antimicrobial drugs available, and this shortage of drugs can lead to under-dosing.

Although antimicrobial resistance is a current and serious problem in healthcare settings, this is only the tip of the iceberg. We are beginning to witness resistance to community-acquired infections. *Streptococcus pneumoniae* is one of the more common community-acquired bacteria, causing a range of diseases including pneumonia, meningitis, otitis media and sinusitis. In the US, about 15 per cent of pneumococcal isolates are resistant to penicillin. Rates are lower in countries which have traditionally been conservative with their antimicrobial use, such as the Netherlands and Germany, and higher in countries that have been more liberal, such as France and Greece. In Spain, resistance rates of 45 per cent have been reported.

Fluoroquinolones are another group of antibacterial drugs that are used for a number of common infections, including bacterial gastroenteritis and urinary tract infection. Resistance to fluoroquinolones by campylobacter – a cause of gastroenteritis – is being reported worldwide, including examples of treatment failure. In the Netherlands, for example, the examination of human faeces reported a three-fold increase from around 10 to 30 per cent over a twelve-month period. Infection with E. coli is responsible for more than 80 per cent of cases of urinary tract infection in young women, with several studies reporting resistance to fluoroquinolones as a first-line treatment.

Increased international travel means that individuals infected with resistant microbes in one country can spread them to another country very quickly. The international spread of antimicrobial resistance is reflected in the recent convention of naming new types of antibacterial-destroying enzymes of a particular class, known as the metallo beta-lactamases, which are capable of destroying a wide range of antimicrobials, after the place where they are first identified. These enzymes confer resistance against the powerful carbapenems, among others, which represent one of our last effective defences against multi-resistant strains of bacteria like *Klebsiella pneumoniae* and E. coli. These enzymes can be spread between different types of bacteria, because the genes that allow bacteria to produce them are contained on plasmids. Recently identified forms of this type of resistance include New-Delhi metallo beta-lactamase (NDM-1), Sao Paulo metallo beta-lactamase (SPM) and Verona Imipenemase (VIM). The UK patient in whom NDM-1 resistance was first identified contracted the resistant strain through travel to New Delhi, where he was hospitalized and first started showing symptoms. There is separate evidence that the NDM-1 resistance was already circulating in India in 2007. The NDM enzyme has now also been reported in Australia, the USA, the Netherlands, France, Sweden and Canada, with most patients having had prior hospital contact in the Indian subcontinent.

Inappropriate or suboptimal use of antimicrobials, such as the use of drugs that are not effective against the microbes causing disease, or patients not completing or missing doses, can promote the development of resistant microbes. Likewise, counterfeit medicines that contain low doses of antimicrobials are also a major cause of resistance. If an antimicrobial is ineffective against a particular bacterium or is only present at levels that do not kill or prevent the growth of the bacteria, those bacteria can continue to multiply, with the chance that the random mutations that can occur at each cell division will make the bacterium resistant and as a result those particular bacteria will grow faster than others while the antimicrobial drug is still in the patient's tissues.

The rapid rate of multiplication among bacteria contributes significantly to the speed of the development of antibacterial resistance, since each division represents an opportunity for mutations to occur in its genetic code. The result of which could be the development of resistance to an antimicrobial drug. When such mutations occur, the bacterium, and the generations that it then gives rise to, have an enormous competitive advantage if exposed to antimicrobial treatment. They will rapidly replace the susceptible strains to become the predominant form within the overall bacterial population. This is a classic example of natural selection of the 'fittest' members of the population, as described by Darwin in his theory of evolution.

Repeated use of antimicrobials also increases the chances that some of the many harmless bacteria that we carry around with us will develop resistance as a result of random mutations. Once resistance has developed in this way, the repeated use of these antimicrobial drugs exerts a selective pressure that favours the survival of the resistant bacteria over those that are susceptible to the antimicrobial. Repeated courses of antimicrobial therapy will also favour the flourishing of commensals ('healthy bacteria' which live in the body) that might already carry plasmids with genes that confer resistance. Under the selective pressure of repeated courses of antimicrobial drugs, these resistant strains become dominant in the microflora that we carry, posing a significant threat. This threat can be realized through the spread of these bacteria to parts of the body where they can cause disease, such as can occur after surgery or serious injury, when the body's normal barriers to the spread of microbes are breached. But they can also arise when the body's normal immunity is reduced as a result of disease (e.g. certain forms of cancer and diabetes) or medical treatment (e.g. high doses of steroids), or when the resistance is transferred to more harmful bacteria through the exchange of plasmids.

The consequences of this for human health are not only that the infection in the person receiving treatment will persist, but also that they pose a risk to others for developing resistant infection, particularly if the form of disease gives rise to symptoms such as coughing or diarrhoea. Taking an average generation time of twelve to twenty-four hours, any single bacterium that is present at the beginning of a seven-day course of antimicrobial treatment has the potential to give rise to as many as 16,000 potential mutation events or, if already resistant, 16,000 resistant 'offspring' during that course of treatment. This many bacteria would pose a significant threat to others if the patient had symptoms such as diarrhoea, with an associated outpouring of the microbe causing the symptoms.

Many of the antimicrobials employed in farming and other non-human uses can also promote resistance in bacteria common to both humans and animals. Bacteria found in animals, including bacteria that cause no significant illness in the animals that harbour them, can give rise to disease in humans. Examples include salmonellas and strains of E. coli that can cause severe bloody diarrhoea and renal failure in humans (verocytotoxin-producing E. coli). The use of antimicrobials to treat animal infections, or as 'growth promoters', can give rise to resistance in the bacteria in those animals that can then be spread to humans.

There are clear links between the development of resistance in bacteria causing infection in animals and the emergence of those strains as a cause of infections in humans. There is evidence that occupational exposure to animals is associated with an increased risk of carrying MRSA on the skin or other parts of the body, with studies showing that MRSA can be found on 10 per cent of equine veterinarians and 18 per cent of small-animal hospital personnel, compared with up to 5 per cent in the general population. It is also known that dogs and cats can carry MRSA, and that in the UK the majority of MRSA strains identified in cats and dogs are those that are commonly associated with human infection. This raises the question of whether we should treat companion animals at the same time as their owners when the latter are found to have MRSA-related disease.

Further evidence for the link between bacterial resistance in animals and humans comes from the Netherlands. Since the discovery of a new strain of MRSA (ST398) in pigs in the Netherlands in 2003, the Dutch authorities have carried out screening of individuals in close contact with pigs and cattle, and through this have found carriage levels of the pig-associated MRSA strain rising from 0 per cent to 33 per cent of all reported MRSA cases in the human population between 2003 and early 2007, particularly among staff working in close contact with pigs and cattle, such as farmers. The pig-associated strain has not yet been encountered in the UK, other than a very few sporadic isolated cases, for which there was no apparent contact with livestock animals.

Worryingly, the threat of resistance might not only come from the use of antimicrobials in humans and animals. The European Centre for Disease Prevention and Control (ECDC) recently published a threat assessment that highlighted possible links between the use of fungicides to prevent the development of moulds on crops and stored cereals and the increase in a particular form of antimicrobial resistance in a fungus (*Aspergillus*) that can give rise to serious infections in humans. Azole fungicides are widely used in Europe to protect crops from disease, ensure yields and prevent fungal contamination of produce, for example in cereals and soybean crops. Although there is no definitive evidence that resistance in human strains has derived directly from plant strains, the ECDC report concludes that 'Given the high frequencies of allergies and asthma, the aging population, the attendant increase in cancers and their treatment and the expanding indications for transplantation, the numbers of patients at risk of developing aspergillosis looks set to rise relentlessly. Although the threat is evident, at the moment we can only provide an educated guess as to the extent of the danger involved. Hard facts are required . . .'

But it is the re-emergence in the West of classic diseases such as tuberculosis (TB) that foreshadows the global threat of antimicrobial resistance. As in many developed countries, in the UK TB was a major cause of morbidity and mortality throughout the eighteenth and nineteenth centuries and declined during the twentieth century until the late 1980s. Since then, incidence has been on the rise. Between 2000 and 2011, over 86,000 individuals were diagnosed with tuberculosis in the UK. The majority of cases come from the more deprived communities within the UK, with the highest burden on migrants coming from South Asia and sub-Saharan Africa. TB is typically treated with a six-month course of different antibacterial drugs. Due to the length of the treatment and the combination of different drugs, it is relatively easy for treatment not to be completed. Unfortunately, TB bacteria that have acquired resistance to the antibacterials used in its treatment are now globally widespread and are being spread from person to person in the same way as drug-sensitive TB. In other words, the drugs don't work. In the UK, cases of TB that are multidrug-resistant increased from thirty in 2000 to over eighty in 2011 and, to date, there have been twenty-four cases with extensive drug resistance. A multi-resistant strain of TB is immune to two of the four most powerful anti-TB drugs, isoniazid and rifampicin. Extensive drug resistance occurs when there is also resistance to any of the fluoroquinolones (such as ofloxacin or moxifloxacin) and to at least one of three injectable second-line drugs (amikacin, capreomycin or kanamycin). Multi- and extensively drug-resistant strains of TB take substantially longer to treat than the ordinary (drug-susceptible) strain, and require the use of second-line anti-TB drugs, which are more expensive and have more side effects than the first-line drugs used for drug-susceptible TB.

The rise of multi- and extensively drug-resistant TB is a global issue. Worldwide, in 2010, over 1 million people died of TB. The global incidence of multidrug-resistant TB was estimated to be about half a million people in 2007 – accounting for about 1 in 20 new cases. So far, extensively drug-resistant

TB is rare. Although it is difficult to be sure, the World Health Organization estimates that about 10 per cent of drug-resistant TB cases are of the extensive form. About 60 per cent of drug-resistant TB cases occurred in Brazil, China, India, the Russian Federation and South Africa. In New York City the number of patients with TB nearly tripled between 1978 and 1992, with a doubling in the proportion with drug-resistant isolates of *Mycobacterium tuberculosis*. About half of patients with multidrug-resistant TB are successfully treated, mainly through directly observed therapy in which healthcare workers watch patients take their medication.

3.
Making the Drugs Work Again

'It is easy to feel overwhelmed and powerless – sceptical that individual efforts can really have an impact. But we need to resist that response, because this crisis will get resolved only if we as individuals take responsibility for it. By educating ourselves and others, by doing our part . . . each of us can make a difference.'

Al Gore, *An Inconvenient Truth* (2006)

Antimicrobial resistance is like climate change in many ways: we are victims of our own success, the science is complicated but compelling, the international politics are fraught with fairness, there is a sense of helplessness, but importantly we can and must do something about it, starting now.

Changing our behaviour

Let us begin with the 'baby steps'. The first preventive measure is to help control the spread of infection. At its simplest, this could mean improved hand-washing. Proper hand-washing with soap and water is the single most important thing you can do to help reduce the spread of infections and help protect you, your family and those around you. The most common way for spreading bugs is by your hands: we have between 2 and 10 million bacteria between fingertip and elbow. As we have seen, most of these bugs are harmless, but some can cause serious illness. We may be inadvertently carrying the bugs that cause diseases such as salmonellosis, MRSA and impetigo – diseases that can be life-threatening, especially for the young and the old. Given that, it is appalling that only 1 in 20 people wash their hands long enough to kill off all infectious bugs after going to the toilet. This is what researchers from Michigan State University in the US recently found out by watching more than 3,700 people washing their hands in bars, restaurants and other public establishments. They also found that 10 per cent of people did not wash their hands and a third did not use soap. In order to kill off the bugs, all it takes is fifteen to twenty seconds of vigorous hand-washing with soap and water – this is about how long it takes to sing 'Happy Birthday to You' twice through.

The second action we can take is to stop demanding antimicrobial medicines, especially antibacterial drugs, from our doctors when we have a viral infection. Worryingly, one in two Europeans believes that antibacterials such as penicillin are effective against colds and flu. They are not. A similar poll in the US reveals the same level of misunderstanding. We need to tackle these misconceptions surrounding antimicrobials. The US Centers for Disease Control and Prevention have been running the annual campaign 'Get Smart: Know When Antibiotics Work' since 1995 with the aim of decreasing demand for antimicrobials among healthy adults and parents of young children. Similarly, in Europe public health advocates have successfully run a number of campaigns to try to reduce the use and misuse of antimicrobials. Since 2002 the French have run the campaign *'Antibiotiques, c'est pas automatique'* (Antibiotics are not automatic). It is aimed at doctors and the public, and has included adverts, Internet campaigns and travelling exhibitions. As a result, there was a drop of about a quarter in the number of antibacterial drugs that were prescribed between 2002 and 2007, with the biggest fall in children. e-Bug is a European-wide Internet-based campaign that aims to educate children of all ages about microbiology, hygiene and the spread, treatment and prevention of disease, including prudent antimicrobial use and how inappropriate use can have an adverse effect on antimicrobial resistance in the community. Its website contains some educational games, including 'Body Busters', where you win by collecting antibacterial drugs to kill off the bacteria but lose if you use them against the viruses.

The threat of antimicrobial resistance is well known to many scientists, doctors and healthcare professionals. But that information has yet to become common knowledge or be translated into meaningful action by us as a society. Part of the reason we don't take the antimicrobial resistance threat seriously is that estimates of current costs are relatively low and future costs, while likely to be high, are hard to predict. It is considered as tomorrow's problem. However, a recent review in the *British Medical Journal* argued that current costs of antimicrobial resistance are misleading and that future costs may have been significantly underestimated. Most of the studies examined did not take into account a world where there are no effective antimicrobials. This included the study with the highest estimated cost of antimicrobial resistance – $55 billion per year for the US – which only looked at the cost of resistance to the health service and lost productivity. The apparent low cost of using antimicrobial drugs today gives us immediate benefit; controlling their use will delay that benefit for tomorrow. This is what economists call a 'hyperbolic discounting'. As a result, an inherent conflict between generations arises. If we continue to misuse antimicrobial drugs, then our children and grandchildren will not benefit from them. The drugs will not work. So in addition to improving our personal hygiene, and stopping demanding antimicrobials from our doctors for the common cold, we all need to raise awareness of the threat of antimicrobial resistance. All of us need to learn about it, explain the threat to our friends and colleagues, and get them to learn about it and explain it to their friends. In this way, we can all help to put antimicrobial resistance into the public consciousness and stop this unfair intergenerational problem in its tracks.

Keep on inventing

One solution to control the threat of antimicrobial resistance is through scientific discovery. An area that is providing some hope is recent advances in the rapid diagnostics of microbes. It is often the case that a doctor will not know the nature of the bug that is causing an infection. In non-life-threatening situations – such as a little girl who has earache – this does not matter too much. The doctor draws on her experience as to what the underlying infection is likely to be, and makes a best guess about the most appropriate antimicrobial to use. If the infection does not subside in two days, she may try a different antimicrobial drug. But in a life-threatening situation a process of trial and error is not good enough.

Consider a young baby boy who is a couple of weeks old. He was born without complications and had been doing well, but suddenly becomes irritable with fever. His parents rush him to Accident and Emergency early one evening. The duty doctors agree that the baby is unwell; he is sluggish and 'not quite right'. As they are not sure what is wrong with him, they suggest that he spends the night in the baby ward, and take some samples that are sent to the hospital laboratory for testing. As a precautionary measure the doctor prescribes cefotaxime, which is a broad-spectrum antibacterial; she is concerned there may be a serious underlying infection but cannot be sure of what is causing it. Using similar techniques to those Alexander Fleming used eighty years ago, the technicians grow some cultures and two days later identify Group B streptococcus (sometimes called GBS) – it takes one day to grow the culture bacteria and another to identify them. The doctor prescribes penicillin for the baby, who recovers with no long-term complications. He is lucky. In the UK around 500 babies a year are infected by GBS and around 50 of them die, and about 1 in 14 have longer-term complications. He is also lucky that his doctors made sure that he was switched to an antibacterial that was likely to be more effective in treating his GBS infection and that would have less of an effect on his helpful commensal bacteria once they knew the cause of the infection.

If techniques can be developed to speed up the diagnosis of GBS and other infections, then this will cut the time it takes for our doctors to prescribe the correct or most appropriate medicine. This in turn will save lives and reduce the risk of further complications. Recent advances in the machines used to sequence DNA mean that it is possible to break the code of bacterial or virus genomes for less than £100. The potential of rapid whole-genome sequencing was illustrated in 2012 by scientists working at the world-famous Sanger Institute in the UK. They used fast genome-sequencing technology to identify, analyse and stop the spread of MRSA in a baby ward at Addenbrooke's Hospital in Cambridge. MRSA is a drug-resistant bug that was involved in 781 and 485 deaths in England and Wales in 2009 and 2010 respectively. A study undertaken in England in 2004/5 found that patients with a bloodstream infection caused by MRSA had a greater than 1 in 3 chance of dying, from any cause, within thirty days of their infection being detected. Using routine screening, staff identified a number of infants who were carrying MRSA, but they were not sure whether they were connected. The Sanger team analysed the genomes of the MRSA samples and found that they were closely related, alerting the authorities to an outbreak that had originated in the baby ward. Although it is still early days and this is very much at the cutting edge of technological development, it is likely that in the near future the immediate identification of pathogens through rapid whole-genome sequencing and other technologies will cut the time it takes to diagnose a microbial infection. This has two benefits: doctors will be able to prescribe the most appropriate drugs, and they will be able to do so more quickly.

The other area where research will matter is in the search for new antimicrobial drugs. There are currently three strategies for discovering new antimicrobial drugs:

1. Systematic testing of the impact of different synthetic and natural substances on the growth of microbes ('whole-cell screening').
2. Identifying specific targets for drugs within a microbe, particularly through the analysis of the whole microbe genome ('target-based screening').
3. Elucidating the three-dimensional structure of potential targets in a microbe (targets identified through genome analysis or identification of existing drug treatment targets) and the development of compounds that might bind and interfere with those structural targets ('structure-based drug discovery').

Much of the history of antimicrobial drug discovery, particularly during the first half of the twentieth century, is one of whole-cell screening, with the first antimicrobial drugs being discovered through the observation of the inhibiting effect that man-made substances (sulphonamides) and naturally occurring substances (penicillin) had on the growth of bacteria in the laboratory.

The earliest antimicrobial drugs to be used widely were the sulphonamides, which are a group of chemical compounds derived from dyes that are manufactured from coal-tar. The discovery of sulphonamides took many years of research by chemists, working in the Bayer company in Germany, who believed that these compounds, which had been shown to be able to bind to bacteria, might be developed to treat infectious disease. After several years of fruitless experiments, the scientists in Germany found a red dye that was effective in treating certain types of bacterial infection in mice. This chemical substance was marketed as Prontosil in the early 1930s, and provided, for the first time, an effective treatment against infections caused by streptococcal bacteria. This was an enormous advance in combating this group of infectious diseases, which included life-threatening bloodstream infections and were a significant cause of maternal death due to puerperal fever.

It was not until sometime after Prontosil had been found to be a successful treatment for infections that it was discovered it was not in fact the dye molecule itself that was effective against the bacteria, but rather a small compound called sulphanilamide, created as a result of the patient's body breaking the dye molecule down. Once this had been recognized, the chase was on among other manufacturers to find other sulpha-containing compounds that could also be used as drugs to treat infectious disease.

As described earlier, the story of the discovery of penicillin is one of the most famous and significant accounts in the history of medicine. For all its significance, and notwithstanding the brilliance of Alexander Fleming in recognizing the importance of what he observed, this discovery was at heart a happy accident. Since this discovery about naturally occurring substances, particularly those produced by microbes themselves as they wage war against each other in their competition for survival, the search for other naturally occurring substances that can selectively inhibit the growth of microbes has been an important part of the strategy for finding new antimicrobial drugs.

In recent decades the search for new medicines by testing the impact of different substances on the growth of microbes has focused on large libraries of synthetic chemical compounds rather than on testing substances produced naturally by microbes, plants or animals. This is, in part, because of a belief that emerged in the 1980s that bacterial resistance might develop less readily to synthetic compounds than to naturally occurring substances. There are also important pragmatic advantages in focusing on synthetic compounds, in that they can often be more readily produced in significant quantities for testing purposes, and their synthesis can be more readily controlled, so that they are less susceptible to being contaminated by other unrecognized substances.

With the failure of screening libraries of synthetic compounds, many of which are now thought to have been unsuitable as sources of compounds with antimicrobial activity, the search is now turning back to naturally occurring substances. With a global microbiome that includes an estimated 5×10^{30} bacteria, the scope for discovering new substances is considerable, as long as the financial and logistical challenges of harvesting these microbes from habitats that include the open ocean and the deepest ocean floors can be met.

The development of techniques that allow the reading of the entire genome (genetic code) of microbes, plants and animals provides new insights into how microbes are made and function, with the potential of identifying new targets for antimicrobial drugs to act against. This genetic information also provides insights into how microbes differ from humans and other animals, which is all-important in the development of drugs that can kill microbes but not harm the cells of the hosts they infect. The first free-living organism to have its entire genome mapped, in 1995, was *Haemophilus*, a bacterium that was a significant cause of meningitis before the introduction of an effective vaccine against it in 1992. Since this landmark event, many other important bacteria causing disease in humans have had their entire genomes sequenced, and as a result over 150 bacterial enzymes that could be exploited by antimicrobial drugs have been identified. While it is encouraging that of these 150 or more potential targets only a small proportion are targeted by existing drugs, it is no easy task finding drugs that can safely exploit the as yet unused targets, and there is a growing sense that the 'genomic revolution' has still to deliver on its early promise. By way of illustration of the problem, over a period of seven years one major pharmaceutical company assessed over 500,000 compounds in sixty-seven screening programmes against potential bacterial targets, at the end of which results for only five of the targets appeared to show any promise, and none of the compounds tested made it as far as being assessed in a clinical trial.

The last, and the newest, of the strategic

approaches to developing new antimicrobial drugs is that of developing 'designer molecules' that can bind to structures within the microbe or its outer wall or coating and as a result inhibit the development or survival of the microbe. This strategy has been made possible by computer applications that enable the three-dimensional structure of microbial cell components to be 'visualized'. Once the structure is understood in this way, it is possible to design molecules that will bind to those structures and so potentially interfere with their normal functioning. To date, the structures of over 600 bacterial proteins have been revealed through this form of computer analysis, opening up new opportunities for drug design, although there are many challenges in moving from an understanding of the three-dimensional structure of a potential target to producing a safe and effective drug that is based on that understanding. A particular challenge is proving to be that of finding antimicrobial molecules that can cross the microbe's wall and remain there in high enough concentrations to have the desired effect. While strategies for designing molecules to improve uptake and retention are known, the chemical characteristics that help with this can, unfortunately, reduce that molecule's ability to bind to the target through which it will exert its effect. This is still a developing science, and one that may lead to the development of new drugs, but the technical challenges, on top of the challenges of taking any new drug to market, do not augur well for a rapid result.

Despite these opportunities, as we have seen in the Appendix no new class of antibacterial has been discovered since 1987. The lack of new drug development is partly because companies can no longer make enough money out of antimicrobials to justify investing in the research needed. It can cost over £1 billion to develop a new medicine, meaning that drug companies are very careful about what areas to research. Currently the return on investment is likely to be much higher for other therapeutic areas, such as cancer, arthritis, diabetes and other chronic diseases. This is because treatment for chronic diseases can last for months or years – as opposed to relatively short courses for antimicrobials – making it more profitable for companies to invest in these new drugs. As a senior executive from a pharmaceutical company put it, 'Without a reliable arsenal of effective antimicrobials, modern medical care will no longer be possible. While the desire to carefully manage the uptake of new drugs is entirely correct, doing so makes it difficult to justify the increasingly high development costs that often run into hundreds of millions of dollars.' Companies are also aware that any new drugs they develop are likely to have a shortened shelf-life as they may be misused and become useless, or that governments will put restriction on their use as a protection against antimicrobial resistance. In short we want new drugs, but we don't want to use them.

The lack of new antibacterial drugs and other antimicrobials is thought by many to be an example of a 'market failure'. Governments often attempt to correct institutional failure through investment and the creation of new incentives, and the same case can be made for the development of new antimicrobial drugs. There are a number of ways that the public and private sectors could work together to make this drug innovation financially attractive. These could be structured around partnership, prizes, prices and patents.

Governments, donors and the private sector already work in partnership to develop new antimicrobial drugs in a number of areas. For example, at the turn of the century the pipeline for antimalarial drugs was non-existent and the old drugs were no longer working due to resistance. Malaria is a mosquito-borne disease caused by a parasite, and was killing 1–2 million people a year, most of them children. Antimicrobial resistance was confirmed in two of the four human malaria parasite species, *Plasmodium falciparum* and *Plasmodium vivax*. But it made no commercial sense for drug companies to invest in new drugs since malaria is a disease most common in the world's poorest countries, whose citizens would not be able to afford the medication. Motivated by this inequity, the Swiss, UK and Dutch governments joined forces with the World Bank and the Rockefeller Foundation to establish the Medicines for Malaria Venture, an example of a Product Development Partnership. The MMV works like a non-profit pharmaceutical company: undertaking discovery and early clinical research. But it does so in collaboration with for-profit companies. In 2009 MMV and Novartis – a drugs company – launched a medicine especially made for children. By the end of 2012, over 171 million treatments of this life-saving therapy had been delivered to more than thirty malaria-endemic countries. The MMV and other similar partnerships offer a potentially new business model for addressing antimicrobial resistance. As the senior pharmaceutical executive suggested, 'To address the rising threat of antimicrobial resistance it's vital that industry and government work together to develop new business models for pathogen-targeted antimicrobials that will encourage investment, reward innovation and create a diverse and robust pipeline of these life-saving medicines.'

In 1795 Napoleon's Society for the Encouragement of Industry offered a prize of 12,000 francs to the first person who came up with a method of food preservation usable by the French military. It was awarded in 1810 to Nicolas Appert, the inventor of food canning. The process utilized heat treatment of food in sealed champagne bottles. In recent years, prizes have been undergoing a renaissance, ranging from a growing number of cash rewards of $10 million or more to an increasingly popular variety of online contests at values of $10,000 or less. The $10 million Ansari XPRIZE was created in 1996 to stimulate a new generation of launch vehicles to carry passengers into space. Meanwhile, only last year, the Automated Student Assessment Prize demonstrated that computers can grade students' essays as accurately as trained human experts. The World Health Organization and the World Bank have proposed the use of prizes for vaccines that would otherwise not be developed or distributed widely enough. A £50 million prize for anyone or any organization that can discover and develop a new class of antimicrobial drugs could shake up research and innovation in the field. Such a prize could be funded by a coalition of governments, foundations and private donors, and would mobilize and focus global talent on a global problem. They would reward the winner by bringing forward and adding to the revenues that the drugs would generate.

The third 'P' is for prices. Drug companies may be tempted to undertake research and development if they were offered an advanced price or market commitment (AMC) for a new type of antimicrobial. Under this approach, the governments or foundations would promise to buy the new drug at a certain price and for a certain number of doses. In exchange, firms would commit to try and develop new drugs, but if they were not successful then clearly they would not get paid. An example is the Pneumococcal AMC, a partnership established in 2009 between the governments of Italy, the UK, Canada, Norway, the Russian Federation, the Bill and Melinda Gates Foundation and the Global Alliance for Vaccines and Immunisation (GAVI Alliance). *Streptococcus pneumoniae* is a bacterium that causes a broad range of infections, including pneumonia and meningitis. It is also the leading vaccine-preventable cause of death in children aged under five worldwide. Nearly 1 million children a year die from pneumococcal infection, the majority occurring in developing countries. In the West a vaccine is widely used; in the UK, for example, it is given to all children under the age of two as part of the national childhood vaccination programme. However, this vaccine is not optimal in developing countries because there are many different strains of the bacteria and specific vaccines need to be tailor-made for different countries. Under the Pneumococcal AMC, the partners pooled funds of over $1.5 billion and guaranteed to buy appropriate vaccines at $3.50 each for ten years. This created an incentive for pharmaceutical companies to invest in vaccine research and development and to expand manufacturing capacity as needed. Although it is too early to assess whether this approach has worked, it provides an interesting model for other antimicrobial drugs.

The final 'P' is for patents. Patents provide an inventor with exclusive rights to their product, typically for twenty years. When a drug company believes it has developed the active ingredient for a new medicine, it will apply for a patent. If granted, this will then allow that company to further develop the medicine for the market. This is particularly important in the pharmaceutical industry, given that it takes about twenty years and about £1 billion to develop a drug. The development time and the patent period will inevitably overlap, giving the company an effective monopoly in selling the new medicine of around eight to twelve years. In this time it is able to recoup its research and development costs and begin to make a profit from its initial investment. Without the exclusive rights provided by a patent to sell a new drug, companies would not make new medicines. One approach that may help persuade companies to develop new antimicrobial drugs would be to extend the patent period from twenty years to, say, twenty-five years. This would act in a similar way as guaranteed prices, as it would secure a revenue stream for the firm – this time for a longer period of time as opposed to a given price.

Conserving our microbial heritage

Even with better hygiene and new and improved drugs we are only buying time. If we don't manage the stock of existing and new antimicrobial drugs well, then the problem of resistance will just keep on repeating itself. We need to recalibrate our relationship to antimicrobials, and we need to do this at a global level. If we do not address this planetary threat, then within a generation we will face an apocalyptic scenario where people will die of routine infections because we have run out of antimicrobial drugs. To avoid going back to the future we must work towards an international framework that would ideally:

1. **Agree to control the use of antimicrobial drugs globally**. This would require the end of over-the-counter sales, the ban of the non-therapeutic use in animals, especially in animal feed, and the prohibition of antimicrobials for non-health reasons.
2. **Provide technical and financial assistance to developing countries in balancing access to essential drugs with action to curb resistance**. This would need to reduce the current high levels of infectious diseases in developing countries and

provide support in controlling and
conserving the use of antimicrobial drugs.

3. **Establish a system to ensure compliance
   with the agreement.** This would
   monitor, verify and enforce an agreed set
   of rules, but also provide early warnings
   of resistant strains of bacteria and other
   microbes and help deter counterfeited and
   substandard drugs.

We need to begin with international agreement
that antimicrobial drugs are a 'common good' that
must be conserved – similar to fish stocks and public waterways. Just as we look after old churches,
beautiful landscapes and endangered animals, we
need to look after our bugs. But as there is no point
in one country or one person doing this on their
own, we need to agree a set of rules to manage
this hidden heritage. There are a number of
approaches that could be adopted, ranging from a
communiqué of signatory countries, a code of
practice sponsored by an existing international
agency such as the United Nations, to more formal
conventions with legal sanction. There are two
broad ways for conserving antimicrobials: limit
the use of microbial drugs through quotas or introduce a price or tax on consumption. Both sound
draconian, but are already widely used in the con-
texts listed in Table 2. None of these schemes are

without their controversies, but they do provide a blueprint for a 'Microbial Manifesto'. With public goodwill and the commitment of our leaders, it is possible to see how these schemes could be used to conserve our antimicrobials. A World Health Organization agreement could limit the use of existing and new antimicrobial drugs for certain diseases and ban their use in agricultural and other products.

Table 2: Examples of international agreements

The UN Framework Convention on Climate Change was originally established in 1992 to cooperatively consider what member states could do to limit average global temperature increases and the resulting climate change. The global response was strengthened in 1997 through the adoption of the **Kyoto Protocol**, which legally binds developed countries to emission-reduction targets. There are 192 parties to the Kyoto Protocol.

The WHO Framework Convention on Tobacco Control is a supranational agreement that seeks 'to protect present and future generations from the devastating health, social, environmental and economic consequences of tobacco consumption and exposure to tobacco smoke' by enacting a set of universal standards stating the dangers of tobacco and limiting its use in all forms worldwide. It came into force in 2005. The treaty's provisions include rules that govern the production, sale, distribution, advertisement and taxation of tobacco.

Table 2: Examples of international agreements

The Convention on the Prohibition of the Development, Production, Stockpiling and Use of Chemical Weapons and on Their Destruction came into force in 1992. By 2013 there were 189 signatories. The main obligation under the convention is the prohibition of the use and production of chemical weapons, as well as the destruction of all chemical weapons. The convention is administered by the independent Organisation for the Prohibition of Chemical Weapons (OPCW). The destruction activities are verified by the OPCW. As of January 2013, around three-quarters of the declared stockpile of chemical weapons had been destroyed.

The European Commission's Common Fisheries Policy (CFP) sets the amount of each type of fish member states are allowed to catch in a certain area, i.e. the total allowable catch (TAC). The CFP was created in 1983 but dates back to 1957 when the Treaty of Rome stated that there should be a common policy for fisheries. The CFP is enforced by member states but overseen by EC inspectors.

G8 Gleneagles Communiqué. In 2005 members of the Group of Eight richest countries in the world agreed to double aid to Africa and to eliminate outstanding debts of the poorest countries. This decision was not legally binding, but was a very public political commitment with oversight provided through continued pressure from society.

The main deal-breaker to these types of agreements will happen when the world's poorer countries point out that the West has benefited from the free and largely unregulated use of anti-microbial drugs for nearly a century. They are likely to suggest that, as with fossil fuel, this key developmental technology is being withheld at the point that their economies are beginning to emerge on the international stage. This is an entirely fair point that should not be contested. As Minister of Health for India, Ghulum Nabi Azad, recently said, 'India is a vast country – our problems are different,' when expressing concerns that curbs on the sale of antimicrobials could hurt vast sections of India's rural populations who don't have access to doctors to prescribe medicines. But no action will also hurt these people. Developing countries face the double whammy of unnecessary deaths from infections and growing antimicrobial resistance. Again, in the past, the international community has provided technical and financial assistance when thinking about these types of global issues. More analogous to the debate on antimicrobial resistance is the World Health Organization's Framework Convention on Tobacco Control. The convention provides assistance to all signatories, but in particular to developing countries, in strengthening national legislations to align with a set of agreed rules that govern the production, sale, distribution, advertising and taxation of tobacco. The convention was signed in 2003, and six years later the 176 countries had established national programmes for the regulation of tobacco, with WHO providing assistance to those countries that could not afford or did not have the experience in implementing such policies.

The existence of suitable monitoring and enforcement mechanisms will be crucial to the success of global strategies to contain antimicrobial resistance. Non-compliance in one country will undermine the efforts made in other countries. But monitoring is not just about enforcement, it will also need to identify bugs that are becoming resistant to our existing drugs and focus on the increasing problem of fraudulent or substandard drugs. The compliance element will need to involve an independent organization that audits how countries implement the agreement, but also provides help and support in that implementation. As such, it will need to act as both a guide dog (helping) and a guard dog (enforcing). Again there are lessons from other treaties. The Organization for Security and Co-operation in Europe observes and assesses elections, but crucially it also engages in the implementation of its own recommendations. Although it has no formal enforcement mechanisms, the combination of openly critical review followed by practical help provides an attractive model for a 'Microbial Manifesto'. It will be important that the remit of a monitoring function is extended to cover the surveillance of emerging strains of drug-resistant infections. This will require a global network that piggybacks on existing national networks, either for collating information on infectious diseases or to expand on activities that have been set up for drug-resistant tuberculosis. At the same time, and as discussed earlier, there will be a need for rapid simple diagnostic tests to identify resistant organisms in animals and humans.

Another important function of a monitoring system could be verifying the quality of drug production. Counterfeit and substandard antimicrobial drugs are dangerous as they do not work and increase resistance. Counterfeit drugs are deliberately fraudulent as they are mislabelled, and have no active ingredient. Substandard drugs are real but do not meet the quality standards set for them. Although we don't know for sure, it is likely that both counterfeit and substandard drugs are more common in low- and middle-income countries with weak or no drug regulation. Anything that is done to reduce the amount of fake drugs in circulation should help to cut the number of people who are ill or dying from infectious diseases. A range of approaches have been developed to tackle counterfeit and substandard drugs, including support for improved manufacturing practices, robust factory inspections, the use of bar codes, electronic tags and other forms of technology to verify a drug's origins, and regulation of on-line sales.

None of these solutions will tackle the problem on its own, but, as with much of the story about the global threat of antimicrobial resistance, each is likely to benefit from international cooperation. This is currently not occurring as countries are hesitant about curbing the use of antimicrobial drugs on their own. In pursuit of perceived national interest, we may all inadvertently become globally worse off. Not only does antimicrobial resistance illustrate the conflict between generations, but also one between individual countries and the international community. In the immediate future the benefit for a country not to address the issue *may* seem greater than the eventual return to all countries in jointly implementing a 'Microbial Manifesto'. But as we have seen, this is not the case. If we don't take collective action, then we will all be responsible for increased disease and death in our children and grandchildren's generations. We know how to fix the global threat of antimicrobial resistance; now is the time to do so by working together.

Conclusion

'One generation plants the trees, another enjoys the shade.'

Chinese Proverb

It is a bright July day. Mrs Xu has not been counting, but it is her fifteenth day of treatment. It started with a wheeze a week after her son's birthday. She had taken Josh to the theme park with a couple of his school friends. She keeps on going back to that day in her mind – it was full of energy and laughter.

The wheeze turned into a cough, the cough into a sore throat. Her husband, Jon, gave her that look – concerned but untroubled. It happened all the time.

When Josh was born sixteen years ago it wasn't always this way. In the final months of her pregnancy, Mrs Xu was advised to stay indoors to separate herself from her friends and family. When Josh went to nursery, she and Jon were lectured by the Head about how irresponsible it was to send a child into public with even mild symptoms. They were given a home testing kit. He spat on a strip of paper. If it turned green he could attend; if it was red he must stay at home. They called the test 'the red spot'. Jon's mum likened it to a pregnancy test.

A few years later, shortly after Josh joined primary school, the global threat was over. Infectious diseases were declining; poor personal hygiene became a thing of the past. The wonder drugs worked again. But this time, everyone understood the miracle.

Mrs Xu recuperated at home. She spent two weeks with her family. Jon and Josh cooked her meals every day and they ate together in the evenings.

She speaks to the doctor. He says she can stop taking the medication. She is well.

The year is 2043.

Appendix

Major classes of antibacterial agents and their use

ANTIBACTERIAL CLASS AND MAJOR EXAMPLES	YEAR INTRODUCED	USE AND STATUS OF RESISTANCE
Sulphonamides sulphamethoxazole sulphadiazine	1932	Widespread development of resistance means that use is now limited to cases of urinary tract infection and exacerbations of chronic bronchitis where there is good laboratory evidence that the bacterial cause is sensitive. They also remain the drug of choice (in combination with trimethoprim – see below) for treating pneumocystis pneumonia.

(continued)

ANTIBACTERIAL CLASS AND MAJOR EXAMPLES	YEAR INTRODUCED	USE AND STATUS OF RESISTANCE
Penicillins susceptible to β-lactamases penicillin G penicillin V ampicillin amoxycillin ticarcillin piperacillin	1944	Much resistance has accumulated, due largely to β-lactamases. Some resistance overcome by protecting with β-lactamase inhibitors. No new penicillin for 30 years.
Tetracyclines oxytetracycline tigecycline	1945	Used to treat infections caused by a wide range of organisms, but their use is decreasing because resistance has become frequent in many organisms. New analogues (e.g. tigecycline) designed to

ANTIBACTERIAL CLASS AND MAJOR EXAMPLES	YEAR INTRODUCED	USE AND STATUS OF RESISTANCE
		overcome this resistance are used against highly multi-resistant Gram-negative bacteria where treatment options are limited. Resistance has been reported but is uncommon.
Chloramphenicol	1947	Can be used to treat a wide range of infections, but its use is discouraged because of its toxicity for humans. No new analogues have been intro- duced since the 1950s.

(continued)

ANTIBACTERIAL CLASS AND MAJOR EXAMPLES	YEAR INTRODUCED	USE AND STATUS OF RESISTANCE
Aminoglycosides streptomycin gentamicin amikacin	1947	Used to treat infections caused by Gram-negative opportunist organisms. A new resistance, which confers resistance to all aminoglycosides, was identified in 2002. Aminoglycosides are toxic to humans and serum levels must be monitored carefully. No new analogues have been introduced since the early 1970s.
Isoniazid	1952	Used to treat tuberculosis. Resistance has been increasing in UK (7.3 per cent of TB cases in 2011), and is commoner elsewhere.

ANTIBACTERIAL CLASS AND MAJOR EXAMPLES	YEAR INTRODUCED	USE AND STATUS OF RESISTANCE
Macrolides erythromycin azithromycin clarithromycin roxithromycin fidaxomicin	1952	These are used mainly in primary care to treat respiratory tract infections. Resistance is widespread in *Streptococcus pneumoniae*, and is also seen in Group A streptococci, a common bacterial cause of a sore throat. Fidaxomicin, introduced in 2012, is used for the treatment of *Clostridium difficile* infection. Clinical activity is comparable to that of vancomycin, but rate of recurrence is much lower. Resistance has not been seen to date.

(continued)

ANTIBACTERIAL CLASS AND MAJOR EXAMPLES	YEAR INTRODUCED	USE AND STATUS OF RESISTANCE
Glycopeptides vancomycin teicoplanin	1956	These had been the 'drugs of last resort' for many years for treating infections caused by Gram-positive bacteria including staphylococci, streptococci and enterococci that are resistant to all other antibacterial agents. Resistance was thought to be impossible, but has emerged and spread in enterococci, and has also been found in *Staphylococcus aureus* (including MRSA strains).

ANTIBACTERIAL CLASS AND MAJOR EXAMPLES	YEAR INTRODUCED	USE AND STATUS OF RESISTANCE
Penicillin resistant to β-lactamase methicillin flucloxacillin	1960	Used to treat staphylococcal infections, but methicillin-resistant *Staphylococcus aureus* (MRSA) is not sensitive to it and increased steadily during the last two decades of the twentieth century.
Metronidazole	1960	Used to treat infections caused by anaerobic bacteria. Few reports of resistance, except with *Helicobacter pylori*.

(*continued*)

ANTIBACTERIAL CLASS AND MAJOR EXAMPLES	YEAR INTRODUCED	USE AND STATUS OF RESISTANCE
Rifampicin	1961	Used to treat infections caused by Gram-positive bacteria and mycobacteria. Primary resistance is rare, but emerges readily by mutation during clinical use. No new analogues.
Cephalosporins *(generation)* cephalexin (1st) cefuroxime (2nd) cefotaxime (3rd) ceftazidime (3rd) cefpirome (4th)	1962	Huge family. Successive 'generations' were developed to overcome resistance to previous generations, but resistance is now accumulating to fourth-generation drugs.

ANTIBACTERIAL CLASS AND MAJOR EXAMPLES	YEAR INTRODUCED	USE AND STATUS OF RESISTANCE
Fusidic acid	1962	Used to treat staphylococcal infections. Primary resistance is rare, but resistance due to mutation is acquired readily in clinical use. No new analogues have been introduced since the late 1960s.
Trimethoprim	1969	Used mainly to treat urinary tract infections which are mostly caused by *Escherichia coli*. Resistance is common. No new analogues.

(continued)

ANTIBACTERIAL CLASS AND MAJOR EXAMPLES	YEAR INTRODUCED	USE AND STATUS OF RESISTANCE
Carbapenems meropenem imipenem ertapenem	1975	These are the most powerful β-lactams, and the most recent of the 'drugs of last resort' for treating Gram-negative bacteria, particularly those acquired in hospital, and that are resistant to cephalosporins. More recently produced drugs (e.g. ertapenem) are used for serious community-acquired infections, including those caused by ESBL-producing *Enterobacteriaceae*, but not for

ANTIBACTERIAL CLASS AND MAJOR EXAMPLES	YEAR INTRODUCED	USE AND STATUS OF RESISTANCE
		hospital-acquired infections as they are not active against *Pseudomonas aeruginosa*. Resistance is emerging and increasing.
Penicillins combined with an inhibitor amoxycillin/ clavulanate piperacillin/ tazobactam	1976	β-lactamases are the main cause of resistance to β-lactams, especially penicillins. Inhibitors overcome some, but not all this resistance.

(continued)

ANTIBACTERIAL CLASS AND MAJOR EXAMPLES	YEAR INTRODUCED	USE AND STATUS OF RESISTANCE
Fluoroquinolones ciprofloxacin norfloxacin	1982	Derivatives of nalidixic acid. They have good activity against Gram-negative bacteria, but resistance has been rising sharply in E. coli since 2000, and is also increasing among cases of gonorrhoea. Resistance is common in MRSA.
Mupirocin	1983	Used topically to treat the carriage of MRSA. Resistance is increasing. No new analogues.

ANTIBACTERIAL CLASS AND MAJOR EXAMPLES	YEAR INTRODUCED	USE AND STATUS OF RESISTANCE
Lipopeptides daptomycin	1984 (but only introduced into clinical use in 2006)	Active only against Gram-positive bacteria and used mainly to treat staphylococci (including MRSA). Resistance has been reported in staphylococci and enterococci but remains uncommon. Now, along with the oxazolidinines, the 'drugs of last resort' for Gram-positive infections that are resistant to all other antimicrobials.

(continued)

ANTIBACTERIAL CLASS AND MAJOR EXAMPLES	YEAR INTRODUCED	USE AND STATUS OF RESISTANCE
Oxazolidinines linezolid	1987 (but only introduced into clinical use in 2001)	Active only against Gram-positive bacteria and used to treat staphylococci (including MRSA) and enterococci (including VRE). Resistance reported in enterococci and staphylococci, but remains low.

Updated from: *The Path of Least Resistance*, Standing Medical Advisory Committee, Department of Health, 1998

Further Reading and Websites

Selected source books, reports and papers

Borchgrevink, C. P., Cha, J., and Kim S., 'Hand washing practices in a college town environment', *Journal of Environmental Health* (2013), 75(8), 18–24. Using field observations of 3,749 people, the research identifies potential predictors of hand-washing compliance and suggests that proper hand-washing practices are not being carried out.

Brown, K., *Penicillin Man: Alexander Fleming and the Antibiotic Revolution* (Stroud: Sutton Publishing, 2004). Biography of Fleming by the curator of the Alexander Fleming Laboratory Museum at St Mary's Hospital NHS Trust, London.

Davies, S. C., *Annual Report of the Chief Medical Officer*, Volume Two, 2011, 'Infections and the Rise of antimicrobial resistance' (London: Department of Health, 2013). Available from: http://www.dh.gov.uk/cmo. In-depth review of infectious diseases and antimicrobial resistance by the UK government's principal medical advisor and the professional head of all directors of public health in local government.

European Commission, *Communication from the Commission to the European Parliament and the Council: Action Plan against the Rising Threats from Antimicrobial Resistance*, COM (2011) 748 (Brussels: EC, 2011). Available at: http://ec.europa.eu/dgs/health_consumer/docs/communication_amr_2011_748_en.pdf. The European Commission's policy on antimicrobial resistance.

Goldin, B. R., and Gorbach, S. L., 'Clinical indications for probiotics: an overview', *Clinical Infectious Diseases* (2008), 46, S96–100. Available at: http://cid.oxford-journals.org/content/46/Supplement_2/S96.full. Review of scientific studies that concludes there is strong evidence that probiotics benefit the management of acute and antibacterial-associated diarrhoea, and substantial evidence exists for their having a beneficial effect in atopic eczema.

Goossens, H., and Sprenger, M. J. W., 'Community acquired infections and bacterial resistance', *BMJ* (1998), 317, 654–7. Available at: http://www.ncbi.nlm.nih.gov/pmc/articles/PMC1113837/pdf/654.pdf. Review paper on the frequency of resistance to antimicrobials among community-acquired pathogens and the number of drugs to which they are resistant.

Gore, A., *An Inconvenient Truth: The Planetary Emergency of Global Warming and What We Can Do About It* (London: Bloomsbury Publishing, 2006). Based on the former US Vice President's lecture tour on global warming and released in conjunction with the Oscar-winning film of the same title.

Guarner, F., and Malagelada, J-R., 'Gut flora in health and disease', *Lancet* (2003), 361, 512–19. Review of the scientific evidence of the major functions of the gut microflora. Concludes that probiotics and prebiotics are known to have a role in the prevention or treatment of some diseases.

Haensch, S., Bianucci, R., Signoli, M., et al., 'Distinct clones of Yersinia pestis caused the black death', *PLoS Pathogens* (2010), 6(10): e1001134. Available at: http://www.ncbi.nlm.nih.gov/pmc/articles/PMC2951374/. By combining ancient DNA analyses and protein-specific detection, the authors demonstrate unambiguously that *Y. pestis* caused the 'Black Death'.

Hoffman, S. J., and Røttingen, J-A., 'Assessing implementation mechanisms for an international agreement on research and development for health products', *Bulletin of the World Health Organization* (2012), 90, 854–63. A review of international agreements used to make commitments, administer activities, manage financial contributions, make decisions and monitor compliance.

House of Lords Select Committee on Science and Technology, *Seventh Report, Session 1997–98: Resistance to Antibiotics and Other Antimicrobial Agents* (London: House of Lords, 1998). Enquiry by their Lordships that concludes that resistance to antibacterial and other anti-infective agents constitutes a major threat to public health, and ought to be recognized as such.

Institute for Health Metrics and Evaluation (IHME), *The Global Burden of Disease: Generating Evidence, Guiding Policy* (Seattle: IHME, 2013). Available at: http://www.healthmetricsandevaluation.org/gbd. This report was based on seven papers published in the *Lancet*, 13 December 2012, p. 380; available at: http://www.thelancet.com/themed/global-burden-of-disease. The global burden of disease (GBD) enterprise dates back to the early 1990s and the most recent iteration of the project is published by the Institute for Health Metrics and Evaluation. See WHO (2008) for earlier iteration.

Krämer, A., Kretzschmar, M., and Krickeberg, K., *Modern Infectious Disease Epidemiology: Concepts, Methods, Mathematical Models and Public Health* (New York: London, 2010). Available at: http://link.springer.com/book/10.1007/978-0-387-93835-6/page/1. Textbook on infectious diseases that provides context and general methods for studying infectious diseases as well as details of transmission routes for specific diseases.

Llor, C., and Cots, J. M., 'The sale of antibiotics without prescription in pharmacies in Catalonia, Spain', *Clinical Infectious Diseases* (2009), 48, 1345–9. Innovative paper that uses actors to assess non-prescription sale of antibacterials in Spain.

McKeown, T., Record, R. G., and Turner, D., 'An interpretation of the decline of mortality in England and

Wales during the twentieth century', *Population Studies* (1975), 29(3), 391–422. An assessment of the contribution that different causes of death make to the mortality decline between 1901 and 1971.

McNulty, C. A. M., Boyle, P., Nichols, T., Clappison, D. P, and Davey, P., 'Antimicrobial drugs in the home, United Kingdom', *Emerging Infectious Diseases* (2006), 12(10), 1523–6. Available at: http://www.ncbi.nlm. nih.gov/pmc/articles/PMC3290930/. A representative survey of UK households that showed that 6 per cent had leftover antimicrobial drugs and 4 per cent had standby antimicrobial drugs.

Mahoney, R., 'Product Development Partnerships: Case studies of a new mechanism for health technology innovation', *Health Research Policy and Systems* (2011), 9, 33. Available at: http://www.health-policy-systems.com/content/9/1/33. PDPs are a form of public–private partnerships that focus on health technology development. The paper examines four case studies of PDPs and shows how they have addressed the six determinants to achieve success.

Mestre-Ferrandiz, J., Sussex, J., and Towse, A., *The R&D Costs of a New Medicine* (London: Office of Health Economics, 2012). Available at: http://www.ohe.org/ publications/. A comprehensive review of how much it costs and the time it takes to research and develop a successful new medicine.

Sharma, P., and Towse, A., *New drugs to Tackle Antimicrobial Resistance: Analysis of EU Policy Options* (London:

Office of Health Economics, 2012). Available at: http://www.ohe.org/publications/. An assessment of the ways in which market failure can be addressed, including examination of the economic impact of different push-and-pull incentives on the net present value of antibacterial R&D.

Standing Medical Advisory Committee, Sub Group on Antimicrobial Resistance, *The Path of Least Resistance* (London: Department of Health, 1998). Available at: http://antibiotic-action.com/wp-content/uploads/2011/07/Standing-Medical-Advisory-Committee-The-path-of-least-resistance-1998.pdf. A review commissioned by a previous chief medical officer, Sir Kenneth Calman, on the issue of antimicrobial resistance in relation to clinical prescribing practice.

Taubenberger, J. K., and Morens, D. M., '1918 influenza: The mother of all pandemics', *Emerging Infectious Diseases* (2006), 12 (1), 15–22. Available at: http://www.cdc.gov/eid/article/12/1/pdfs/05-0979.pdf. Review of the 'Spanish' influenza pandemic of 1918–19, which caused approximately 50 million deaths worldwide and remains an ominous warning to public health.

Whitman W. B., Coleman, D. C., and Wiebe W. J., 'Prokaryotes: The unseen majority', *Proceedings of the National Academy of Science* (1998), 95, 6578–83. Available at: http://www.pnas.org/content/95/12/6578.full. An attempt to estimate the number of prokaryotes on Earth through the examination of several representative habitats.

World Health Organization (WHO), *The Global Burden of Disease: 2004 Update* (Geneva: World Health Organization, 2008). Available at: http://www.who.int/topics/global_burden_of_disease/. The WHO global burden of disease (GBD) measures burden of disease using the disability-adjusted life year (DALY). The DALY metric was developed in the original GBD 1990 study to assess the burden of disease consistently across diseases, risk factors and regions. See IHME (2013) for subsequent iteration.

World Health Organization (WHO), *World Health Statistics, 2011* (Geneva: World Health Organization, 2011). Available at: http://www.who.int/whosis/whostat/2011/en/. The WHO's annual compilation of health-related data for its 193 member states, including a summary of the progress made towards achieving the health-related Millennium Development Goals (MDGs) and associated targets.

Useful websites

e-Bug is a free educational resource for classroom and home use, and makes learning about microorganisms, and the spread, prevention and treatment of infection, fun and accessible for all students. http://www.e-bug.eu/

Wash Your Hands . . . Give Soap a Chance is a NHS hand-washing campaign that aims to improve hand hygiene. http://www.wash-hands.com/

European Surveillance of Antimicrobial Consumption Network (ESAC-Net) is a Europe-wide network of national surveillance systems, providing European reference data on antimicrobial consumption. ESAC-Net collects and analyses data on antimicrobial consumption from EU and EEA/EFTA countries, both in the community and in the hospital sector. http://www.ecdc.europa.eu/en/activities/surveillance/esac-net/pages/index.aspx

Multidrug-resistant tuberculosis (MDR-TB) is a website maintained by the World Health Organization (WHO) that provides information on the major public health problem that threatens progress made in TB care and control worldwide. http://www.who.int/tb/challenges/mdr/en/index.html

Acknowledgements

We would like to thank and acknowledge everyone who has supported us in writing this book. Needless to say, their input, advice and comments have been essential to this endeavour, but any errors or misunderstandings are solely ours. We are particularly grateful to the assistance given by: Ben Brusey, Joanna Chataway, Jeremy Grant, Sarah Hopwood, Simon Howard, Deepa Jahagirdar, Alan Johnson, Jorge Mestre-Ferrandiz, Ellen Nolte, Mafalda Pardal, Emma Pitchforth, Jennifer Rubin, Lucila Sanz and Jirka Taylor.

He just wanted a decent book to read ...

Not too much to ask, is it? It was in 1935 when Allen Lane, Managing Director of Bodley Head Publishers, stood on a platform at Exeter railway station looking for something good to read on his journey back to London. His choice was limited to popular magazines and poor-quality paperbacks – the same choice faced every day by the vast majority of readers, few of whom could afford hardbacks. Lane's disappointment and subsequent anger at the range of books generally available led him to found a company – and change the world.

'We believed in the existence in this country of a vast reading public for intelligent books at a low price, and staked everything on it'
Sir Allen Lane, 1902–1970, founder of Penguin Books

The quality paperback had arrived – and not just in bookshops. Lane was adamant that his Penguins should appear in chain stores and tobacconists, and should cost no more than a packet of cigarettes.

  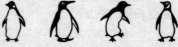

Reading habits (and cigarette prices) have changed since 1935, but Penguin still believes in publishing the best books for everybody to enjoy. We still believe that good design costs no more than bad design, and we still believe that quality books published passionately and responsibly make the world a better place.

So wherever you see the little bird – whether it's on a piece of prize-winning literary fiction or a celebrity autobiography, political tour de force or historical masterpiece, a serial-killer thriller, reference book, world classic or a piece of pure escapism – you can bet that it represents the very best that the genre has to offer.

Whatever you like to read – trust Penguin.